The Good Mommy's Guide to Her Little Boy's Penis

by Adrienne Carmack, MD

This booklet is intended for informational purposes only, and is not a substitute for medical care by a qualified medical practitioner. If you or your child has a health issue, please seek appropriate care.

First Printing: April 2015.

Published by Adrienne Carmack/United States of America.

ISBN 978-0-9903060-3-0

Design and layout: Janet W. Hardy, www.janetwhardy.com.

Acknowledgments

It is with the warmest gratitude that I thank Marilyn Milos, RN, for her kind input into the creation of this booklet. Her lifetime of advocacy for baby boys has shown me the power one gentle soul has to make a huge difference in our world.

Dedicated to all the mommies who have been blessed
with the gift of a little boy to nurture and love

Introduction

Congratulations! And thank you for reading *The Good Mommy's Guide to Her Little Boy's Penis*. I wrote this book because, as a urologist and a mommy, I realized that a new mommy needs help knowing just how to best take care of her little boy's penis. Not all the advice new mommies get is good (as you have realized by now, I'm sure!), and I want to lay out the simple facts so you know how to help your little boy grow up healthy and problem-free.

Most mommies naturally know how to clean their little girls' genitalia. You know which parts are sensitive, which parts need to be washed, and which parts don't. Yet many mommies worry, rightfully so, that they won't know what to do for their little boy and that he may develop problems.

But did you know that taking care of your little boy's penis is actually quite simple? With a clear understanding of the anatomy of the penis, the functions of different parts of the penis, and why and how cleaning affects it, you'll learn the best way to care for your little one.

I hope to raise your confidence so you can avoid the problems that arise when bad advice is given. Enjoy this wonderful time with your new baby boy!

Part 1: *All About Your Baby Boy's Penis*

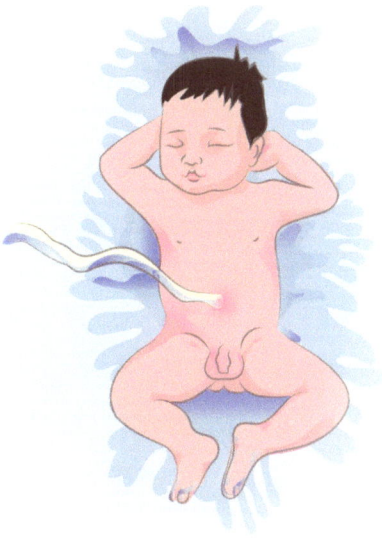

Congratulations on the birth of your baby boy! This is the beginning of a wonderful journey, in which you will come to know, love, and understand this child in the unique and special way that only mommies can. Your little boy will show you new parts of himself as he grows, and you will do a lot of learning along the way!

But, first things first. There is one part of your little boy that you probably don't have much experience with, because most mommies were born without one: his penis. So let's talk about it.

Most baby boys are born with genitals that look like this:

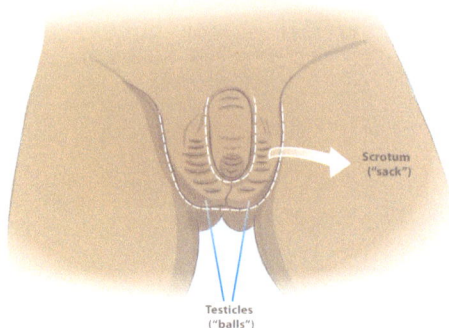

Scrotum
("sack")

Testicles
("balls")

A little boy's genitals include two main parts on the outside—the penis and the scrotum. The scrotum (sometimes called the "sack") holds the two testicles (the "balls"). This anatomical design will eventually help the testicles produce sperm (which travel into the body to become a part of semen).

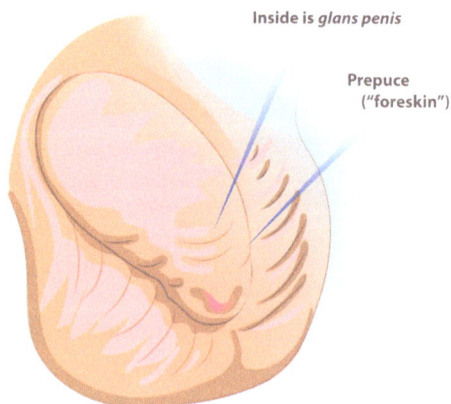

Inside is *glans penis*

Prepuce
("foreskin")

The penis comes with a covering to protect its sensitive head (the glans penis), called the prepuce, or "foreskin."* The foreskin almost always covers the head of the penis at birth. It is attached by healthy tissue similar to that which connects the fingernail to the nail bed.

There are several layers of the foreskin, and the innermost one, the mucosal layer, is the one that is connected to the head of the penis.† The middle layer of the foreskin, the Dartos muscle, helps keep the foreskin closed over the head of the penis in the infant, and, in the man, enlarges during an erection. The outer layer of the foreskin is rich with blood vessels and nerves.

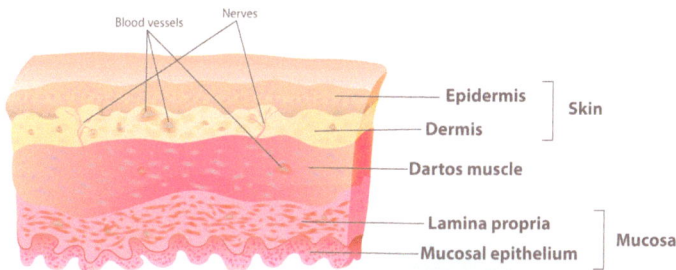

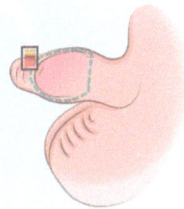

---

* Did you know that girls have a prepuce too? It is commonly called the clitoral hood, and this highly specialized tissue is one of the most sensitive parts of a woman's genitalia.

† Like all mucosal tissue found in the body, the foreskin also contains important immune cells that help defend the body from the outside world.

Over time, the foreskin produces a substance called smegma, which looks like cottage cheese, and this helps the foreskin tissue separate from the tissue on the head of the penis, so that, eventually, the foreskin can retract to allow for sexual function.

Because of these natural attachments, the foreskin is almost always not retractable at birth, so you can't see what's under it. But, in this picture, we'll take a peek right through the foreskin:

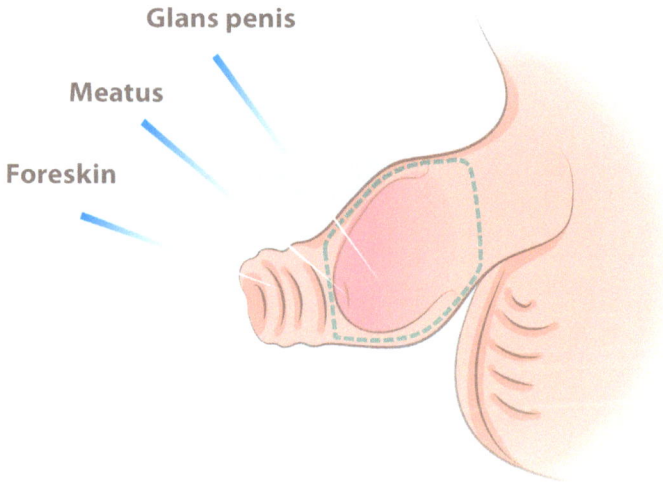

Glans penis

Meatus

Foreskin

Under the foreskin, at the tip of the head of the penis, is the urethral meatus. The urethra is the tube that connects to the bladder and through which urine (pee) comes out. The meatus is the opening at the end of the urethra. The foreskin helps protect the meatus from closing off by keeping it covered and moist.

When a little boy pees, the pee comes out of the meatus and out the opening of the foreskin. As the foreskin attachments to the head of the penis begin to separate naturally as the baby boy grows, sometimes pee fills these new spaces and creates ballooning, which is a normal developmental process that is seen in many little boys.

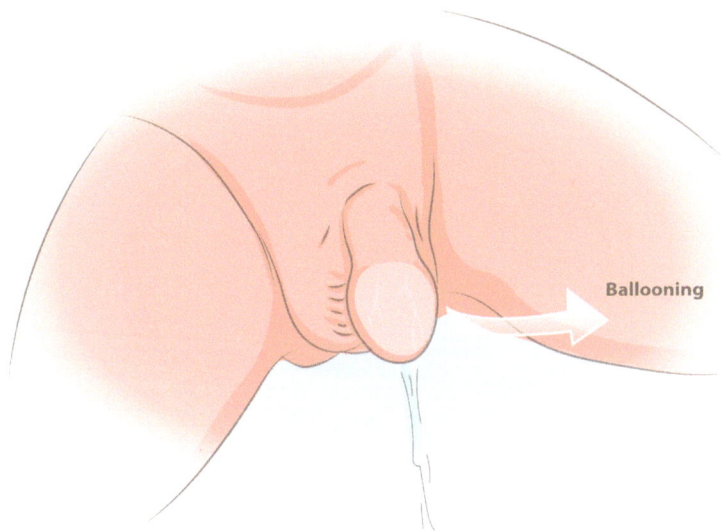

Ballooning

When your little boy becomes a man, his foreskin will serve some very important functions. The foreskin continues to cover the head of the penis in many men when they are not erect, helping to keep this tissue sensitive. It actually contains up to half of the skin of the penis, and, because of its redundancy, stretches out as the penis becomes erect yet is still able to glide smoothly, thus minimizing friction for the man and his partner. During an erection, the foreskin stretches to cover the shaft of the penis, exposing the inner foreskin and the ridged bands that encircle the foreskin opening. These tissues are highly sensitive and erogenous. Because the lining of the foreskin is mucosal tissue, it also produces moisture, which aids in lubrication for the man and his partner during sexual activity. Since the foreskin contains the highest concentration of nerve endings in the entire penis and is the most sensitive part, like the clitoris, it will bring the man to whom it belongs a lot of pleasure.

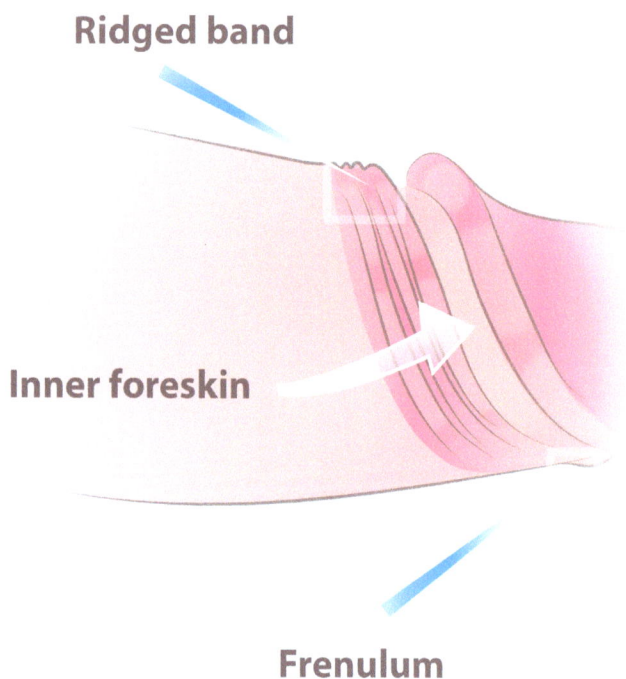

Ridged band

Inner foreskin

Frenulum

Now that you know all about your little boy's parts, let's talk about what you need to do, as his mommy, when he is still so little that he needs your help.

Part 2: Just How Do You Wash It?

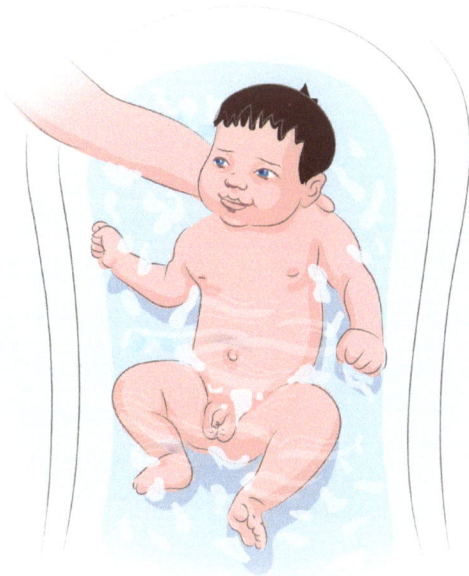

This is a question many, many mommies ask, and, unfortunately, many, many mommies are given incorrect information. As we discussed, the foreskin is attached to the head of the penis in order to protect it. And the inside is lined with mucosal tissue, which is very different from skin.

Think about your eyelid. The outside is sensitive, delicate skin, and the inside is mucosal tissue. It keeps your eyeball moist, protects it, and glides over it easily. The foreskin is very similar to this tissue in many ways, and ought to be cleaned in the same way.

So how do you clean your eyelid? That is how a baby boy's foreskin needs to be cleaned as well.

The outside can be washed along with the rest of the genitals. Like removing sleep from the corner of your eye, any dirt or debris on your son's penis can also be gently wiped away with your finger or a soft rag.

You do not need to use soap to do this on your son's penis any more than you do on your eyelid. Soap irritates mucosal tissue and dries it out. Soap removes the protective functions of the naturally moisturizing mucosal tissue. **Don't wash your baby's foreskin with soap.**[*]

It has become quite common in the United States for doctors, nurses, and other parents to tell mommies that they need to retract their son's foreskin when he bathes. This is not true. As we've already discussed, your son's foreskin is able to separate on its own, with time. There is no need for it to be separated until he becomes sexually active. The foreskin covers the head of the penis for a reason, and when your son's body no longer needs this protection, it will unstick itself naturally. **Do not retract your son's foreskin, and do not allow anyone else to do so.**

---

[*]   If you also have a little girl, you probably already know that you should not wash inside her inner labia and vagina (where mucosal tissue is also found) with soap either.

Retracting the foreskin and applying soap to the delicate mucosal tissue is dangerous. Pulling on this sensitive tissue can cause tearing and lead to infections and scarring. Many boys who need emergency care and even circumcision (removal of the foreskin) do so because of premature retraction of the foreskin by parents or caregivers. Most episodes of foreskin irritation and scarring can be prevented by simply avoiding these practices.

Remember, just rinse the outside of the penis gently, from body to tip, as you would wash a finger. Leave the tissues where they are, and know they are there for a reason.*

---

* Little girls also have tissue that naturally protects their sensitive mucosal tissue. This is called the hymen. Like little boys, as little girls mature and experience sexual functions such as menstruation, intercourse, and childbirth, the hymen naturally opens.

Part 3: Communicating Acceptance

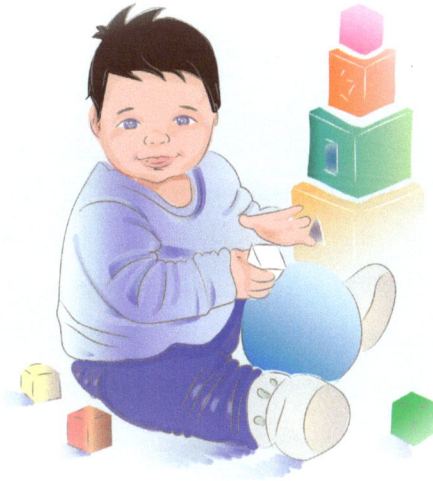

One of the final and most important things you can do to help your child grow up with a positive and healthy body image is to communicate acceptance of his body.

Though of course there are times and places where it is socially appropriate to have the genitals covered, leaving your little boy's penis open to air at least sometimes has many benefits. One of these is that it helps you and him to learn his signals that he needs to pee or poo. In many cultures, babies actually almost never wear diapers, and their mothers rapidly learn to recognize their signals. When their baby needs to eliminate, they hold him over a potty or the ground. This can help potty-training occur earlier. Some call this elimination communication, or natural infant hygiene, and you can find a lot more tips with a quick Internet search. It's worth knowing about to keep your son out of diapers as often as is practical.

As your little boy gets older, he will naturally be drawn to touch his penis, because, well, it feels good. He will begin to pull and tug on his foreskin at some point, if he is allowed to. This is normal, and will actually help the process of foreskin separation in a safe and natural way. Allowing him to touch his own penis when it is appropriate is beneficial. When he gets old enough, you can gently educate him on societal rules and let him know that touching himself is a private activity.

Also, remember to use positive language. When changing diapers or cleaning your child, avoid making foul faces or talking about him being "stinky." As a child gets older, these actions and words can create shame, which does not lead to healthy sexual development. Instead of calling diapers "dirty," consider using more neutral words such as "wet" and describe the next diaper as "dry" or "new" instead of "clean." This will help your child avoid developing the belief that pee, poo, and his genitals are "bad" or "dirty" and instead understand that they are a normal part of life. Social boundaries can still be taught without the adverse consequences of shaming.

Conclusion

Raising a baby boy is a wonderful opportunity! As you see, there is very little you actually need to do to give your child a good start towards a healthy self-image and sexual development. I hope the knowledge shared here has built your confidence to do what is right for your child.

Remember:

- The foreskin is a highly sensitive part of the penis and serves protective functions for all boys, from birth through adulthood.
- Cleanse the delicate foreskin gently. Do not wash your son's foreskin with soap.
- The foreskin is attached to the head of the penis and normally separates naturally and painlessly as he ages. Do not retract your son's foreskin, and do not allow anyone else to do so.
- Allow time out of diapers when feasible. Allow your child to touch his own genitals, and teach him about social appropriateness without shaming.
- Use positive language when changing diapers and helping with pottying.

Further Reading

For more information about the foreskin, visit

- Circumcision Information and Resource Pages at www.cirp.org
- Circumcision Resource Center at www.circumcision.org
- The Whole Network at www.thewholenetwork.org/the-foreskin-and-penis.html
- National Organization of Circumcision Information Resource Centers at www.nocirc.org/publish

For more information about the benefits of diaper-free time, visit diaperfreebaby.org.

For more information about gentle and natural parenting, visit mothering.com.

About the Author

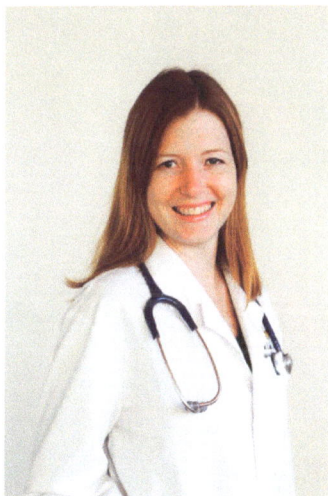

Before she became a mommy, Adrienne became a urologist (this took a lot longer than nine months!). Along her journey, she realized how much knowledge of normal sexuality was lost through the cultural practices of circumcision (popularized in the US in the 1800s to prevent masturbation by reducing pleasure) and modernization (diapers, diapers, oh my!). She wrote this book to bring that knowledge back to new mommies who want to give their sons the best start but are often faced with conflicting information from their well-meaning families, friends, and health care providers.

www.ingramcontent.com/pod-product-compliance
Lightning Source LLC
Chambersburg PA
CBHW041105110426
42740CB00043B/156

* 9 7 8 0 9 9 0 3 0 6 0 3 0 *